Early Bird Stories

Food and You

An Alien's Guide

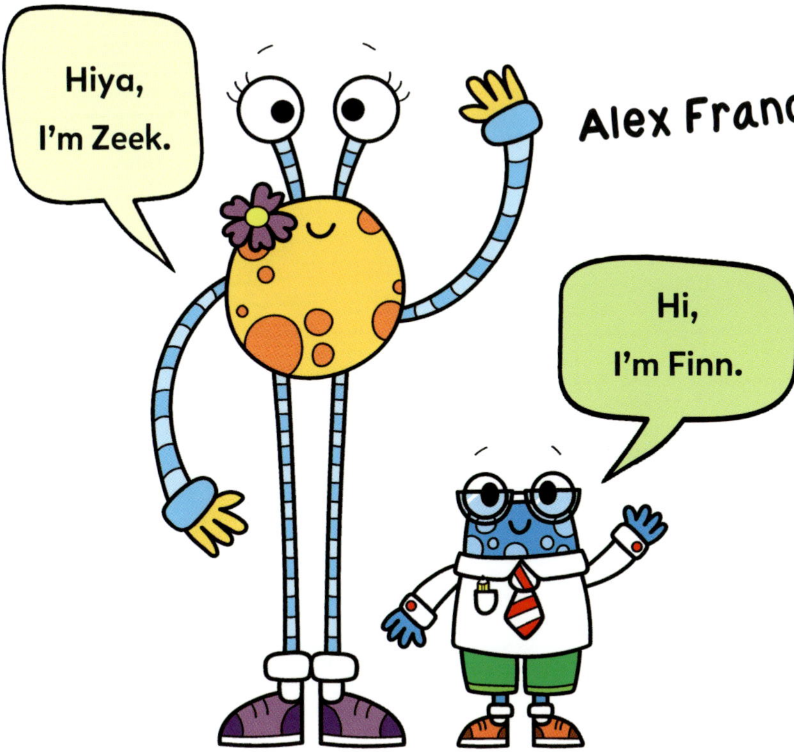

Alex Francis

Early ★ Reader

Lerner Publications ◆ Minneapolis

First American edition published in 2020 by Lerner Publishing Group, Inc.

An original concept by Alex Francis

Illustrated by Alex Francis

First published by Maverick Arts Publishing Limited

Maverick
arts publishing

Licensed Edition
Food and You: An Alien Guide

Lerner Publications Company
An imprint of Lerner Publishing Group, Inc.
241 First Avenue North
Minneapolis, MN 55401 USA

For reading levels and more information, look up this title at www.lernerbooks.com.

Main body text set in Mikado. Typeface provided by HVD Fonts.

Library of Congress Cataloging-in-Publication Data
Names: Francis, Alex, author.
Title: Food and you : an alien's guide / Alex Francis.
Description: First American edition. | Minneapolis : Lerner Publications, 2021. | Series: Early bird nonfiction readers - purple (early bird stories) | Includes index. | Audience: Ages 5–9 | Audience: Grades 2–3 | Summary: "Humans need food to be healthy and have energy. From portion size to vitamins and minerals to water intake, alien tour guides Zeek and Finn explain the basics of food literacy"— Provided by publisher.
Identifiers: LCCN 2020002979 (print) | LCCN 2020002980 (ebook) | ISBN 9781728415062 (library binding) | ISBN 9781728415284 (paperback) | ISBN 9781728415291 (ebook)
Subjects: LCSH: Nutrition—Juvenile literature. | Food—Juvenile literature.
Classification: LCC RA784 .F657 2021 (print) | LCC RA784 (ebook) | DDC 613.2—dc23

LC record available at https://lccn.loc.gov/2020002979
LC ebook record available at https://lccn.loc.gov/2020002980

Manufacured in the United States of America
1-48662-49085-1/21/2020

INCOMING MESSAGE

Dear Finn and Zeek,

We are heading to Earth soon to sample some of its famous food! However, we're not sure what the food will do to our bodies or if it will be bad for us.

Can you please help?

From,
Om and Nom
(Planet Gobble)

Introduction

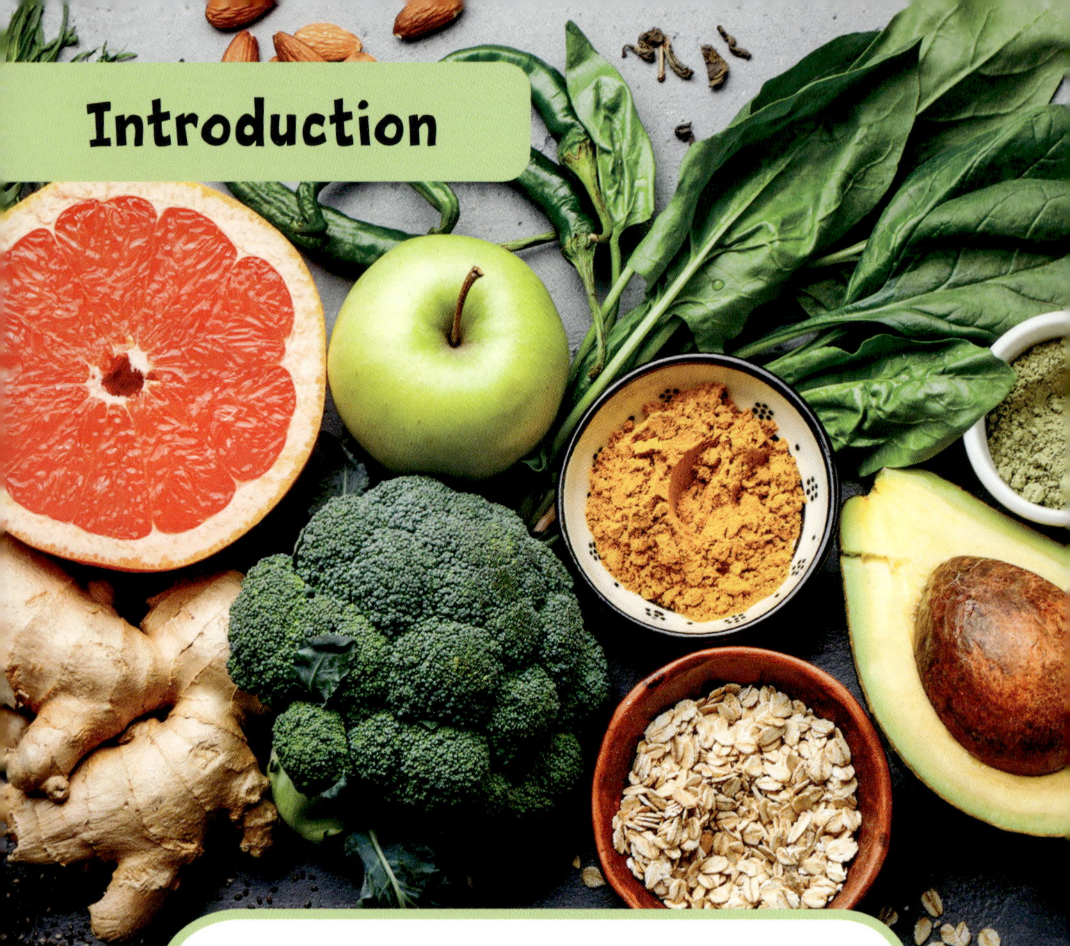

Humans and animals have to eat food to stay healthy. Food helps their bodies grow and work properly. Let's take a look!

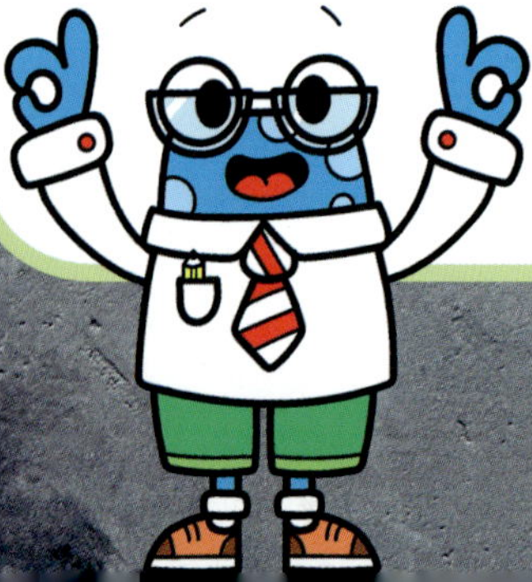

Table of Contents

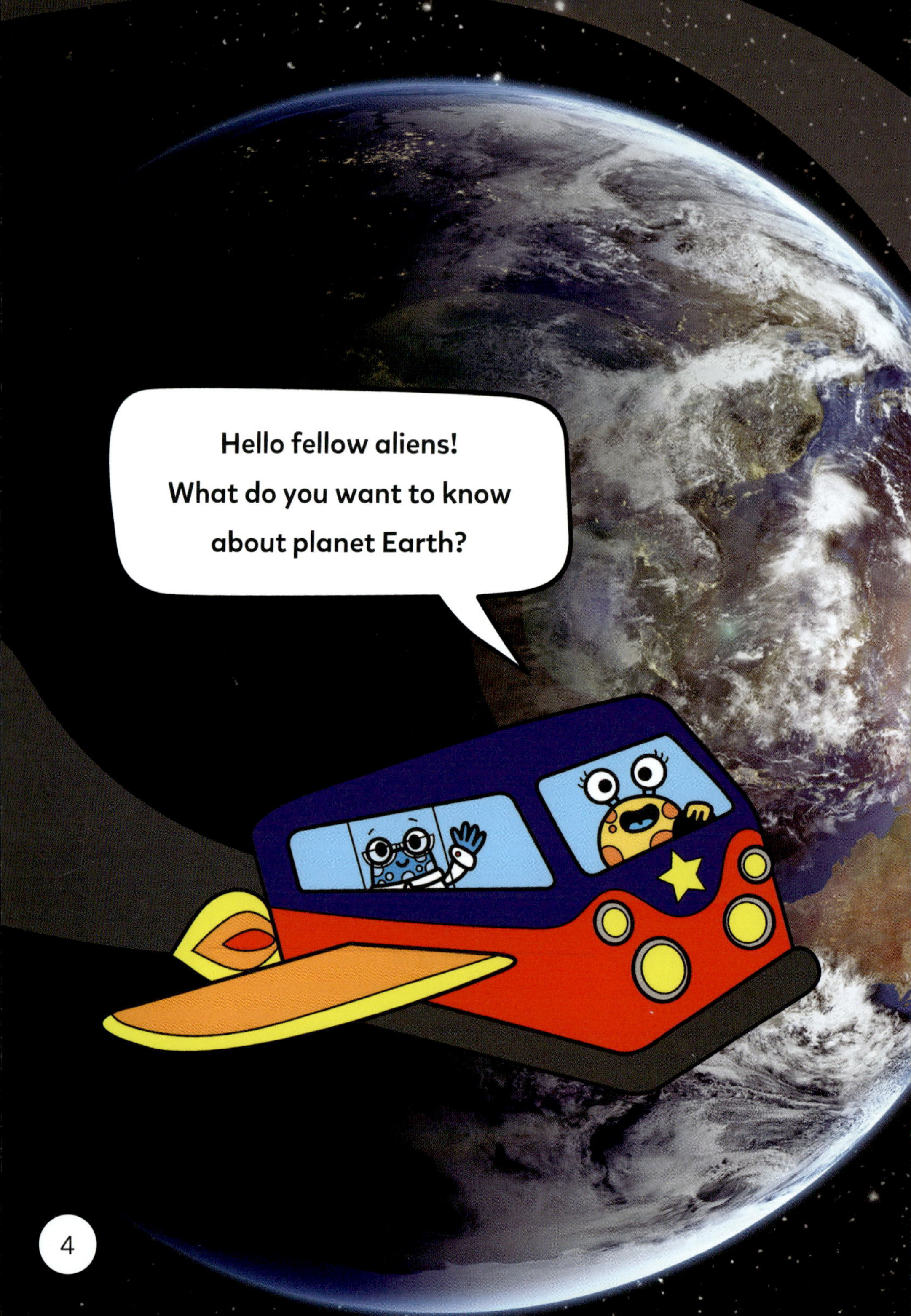
Hello fellow aliens!
What do you want to know
about planet Earth?

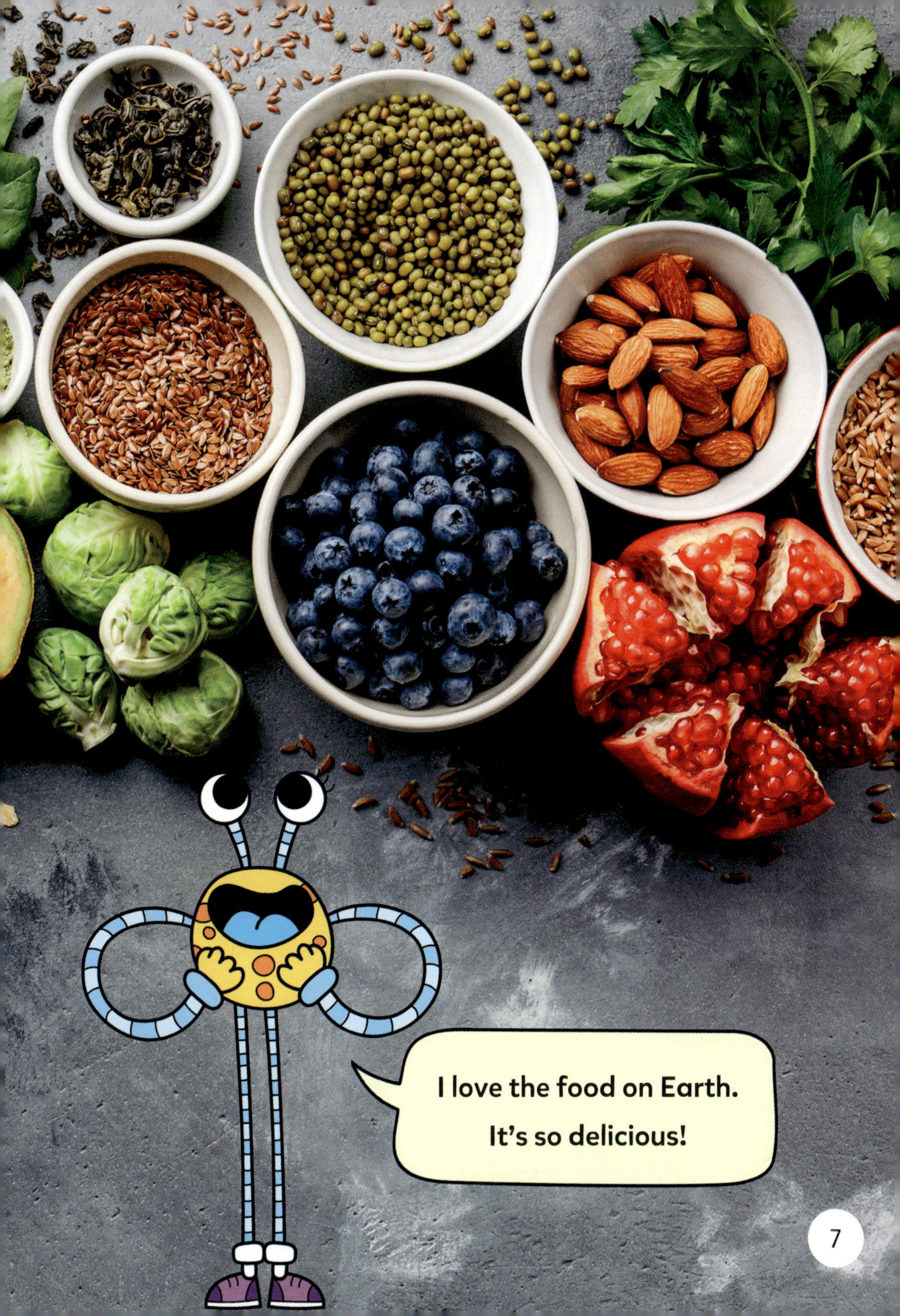
I love the food on Earth.
It's so delicious!

Portion Size

How much food you eat is just as important as what you eat.

Food gives your body **energy.** If you eat too much food, your body can't use all the energy. The extra food gets stored in your body as fat. This means that if you don't exercise enough, you might gain weight.

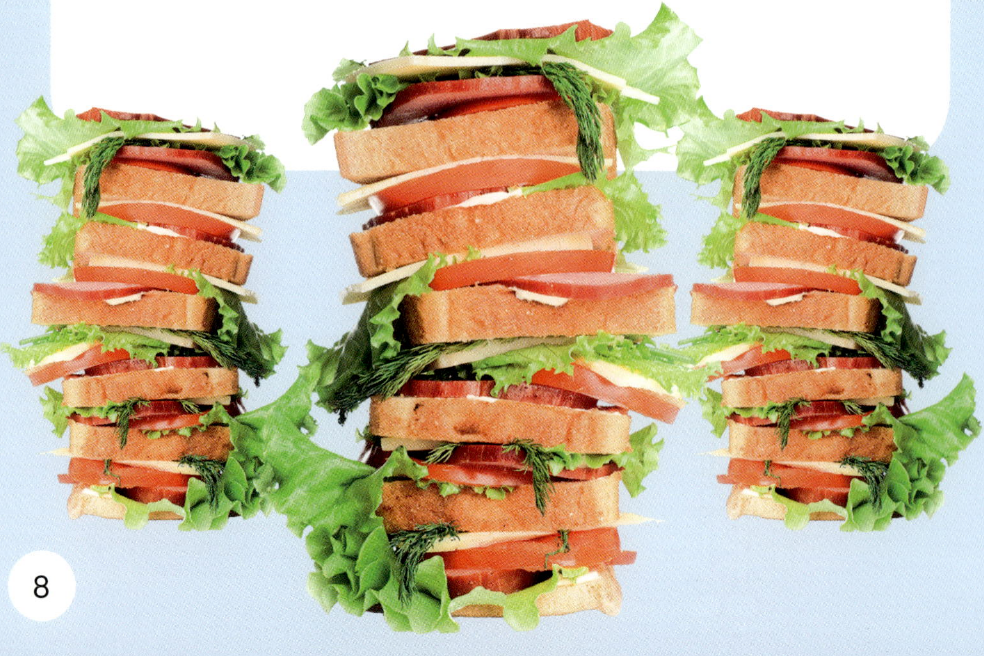

If you eat too little, your body doesn't have enough energy. This means you will feel tired and lose weight.

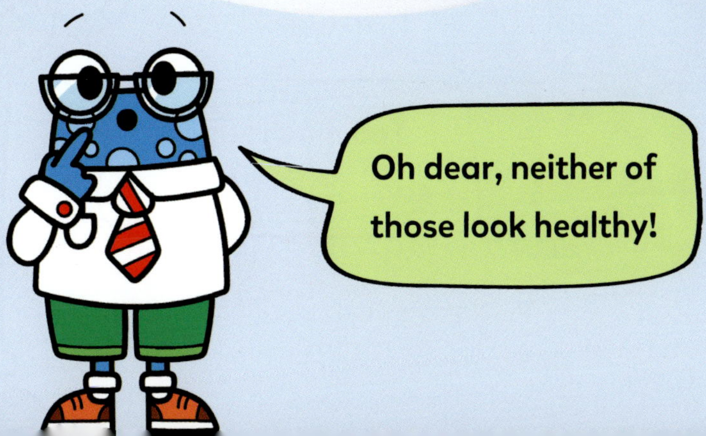

Sugar

A lot of food has sugar in it. Chocolate, candy, ice cream, ketchup, and soda are all foods with lots of sugar.

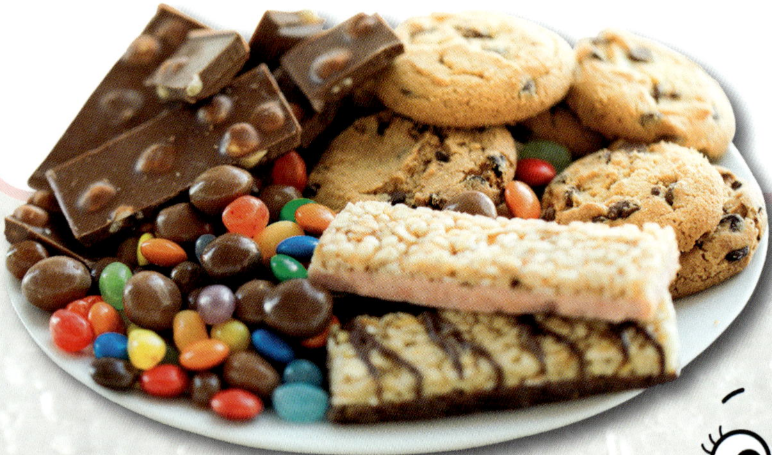

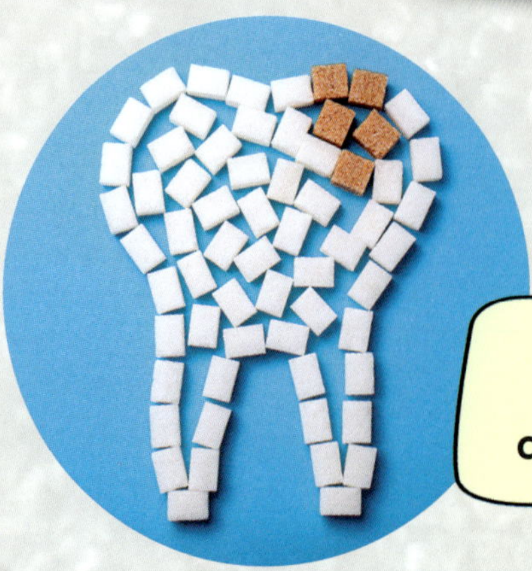

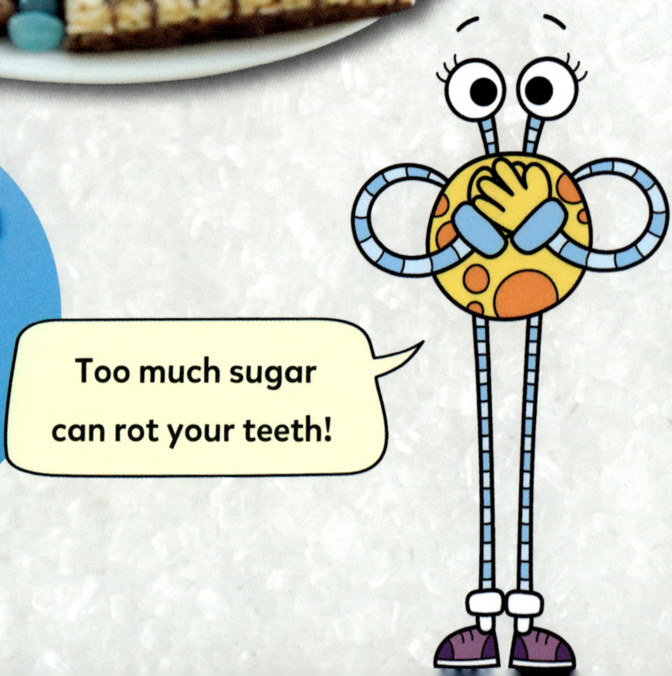

Since your body can use sugar for quick energy, a little bit of sugar is fine. But too much sugar can be bad for you. Too much sugar can cause tiredness, a bad mood, feeling hungrier, bad skin, and an upset stomach.

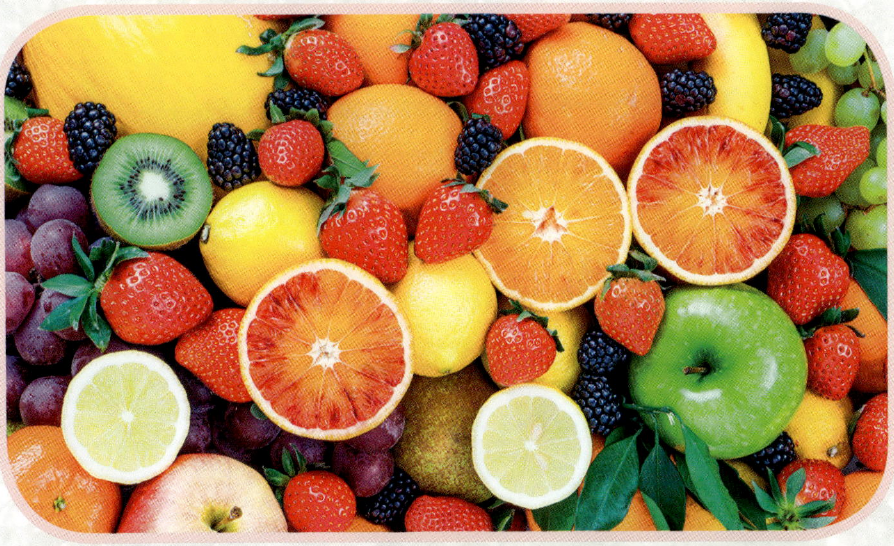

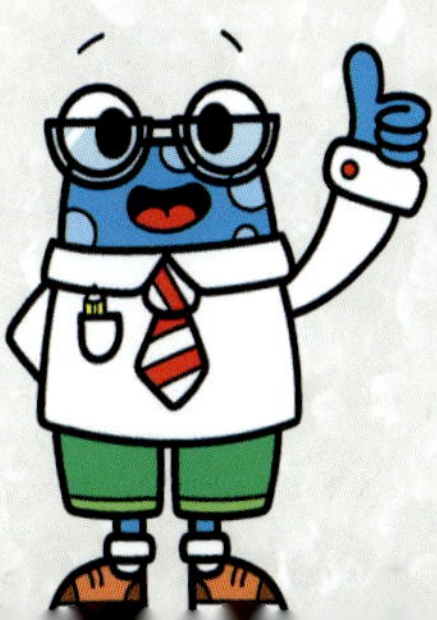

Natural sugar from fruit and other food is better for you because it fuels you for longer.

Fats

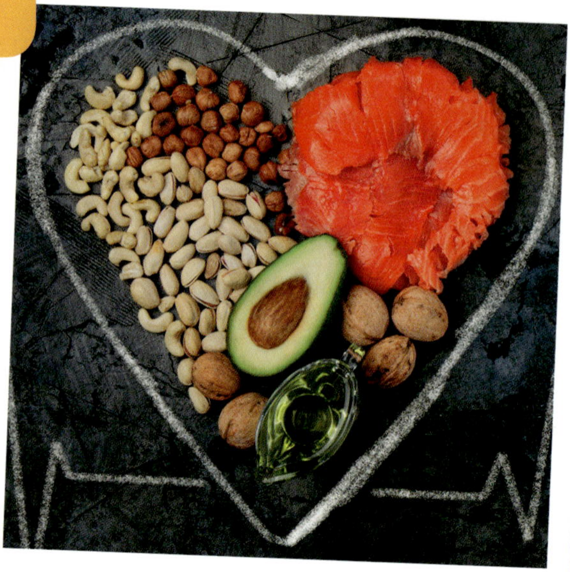

Healthy fats

Everyone needs some fat in their diet, but it's important not to eat too much fat. Some types of fat are better for you than others. For example, peanuts, almonds, olive oil, sunflower oil, avocados, and oily fish all contain fats that are good for you.

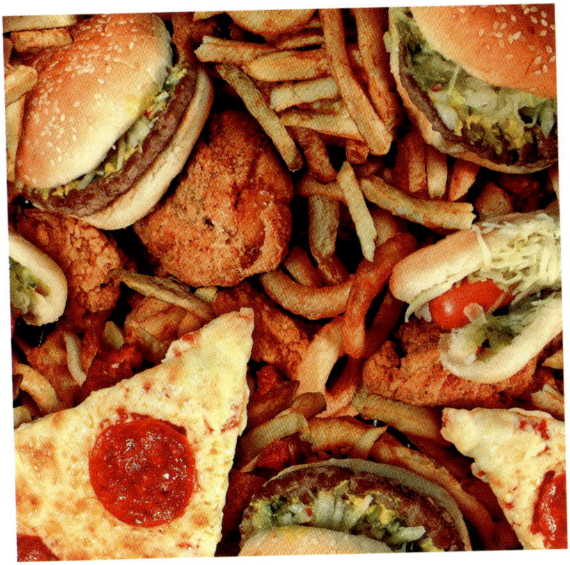

Unhealthy fats

Too much fat is not good for you, so it's important to limit the amount of fried food you eat. Things like fries and chips are fine to eat occasionally but not good to eat every day.

Protein

Meats and fish are main sources of protein, but it is also in eggs, dairy products, beans, nuts, seeds, and more! It is very good for you, so be sure to eat some. But too much protein can upset your liver and kidneys.

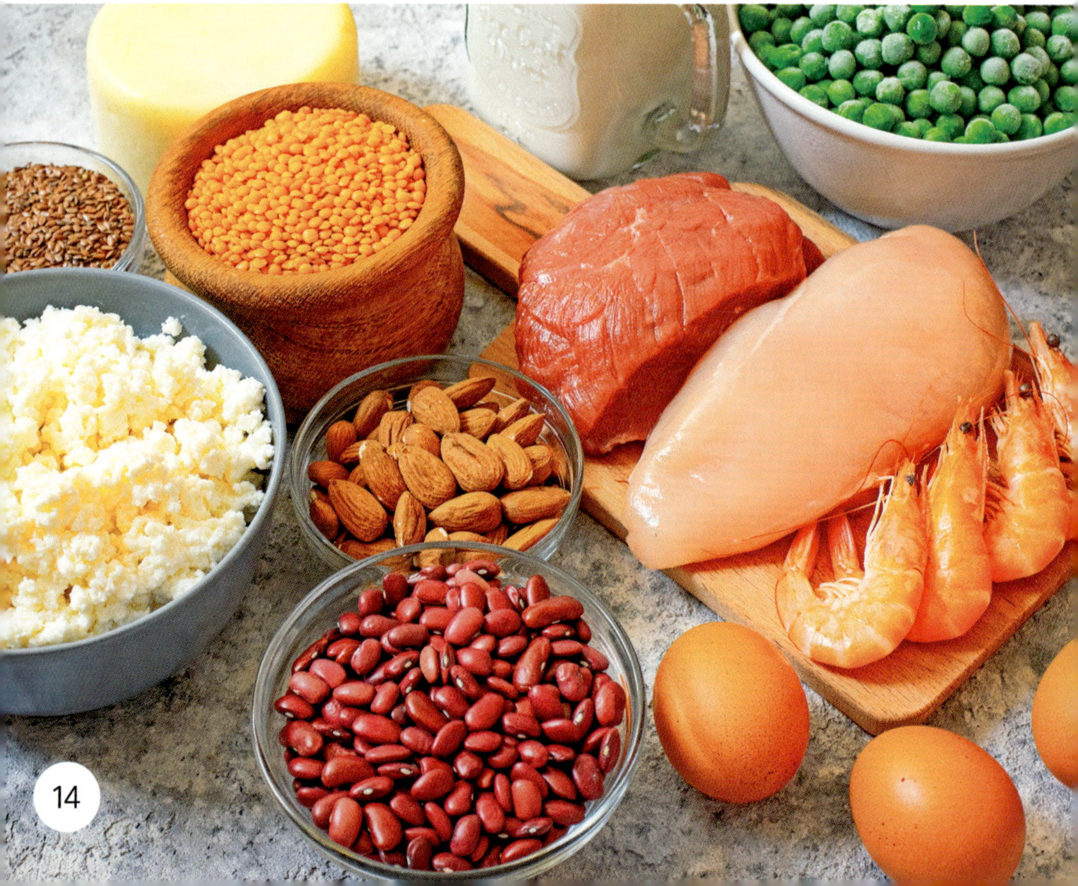

Your body uses protein to build and repair itself, and it is an important building block for bones, muscles, **cartilage**, skin, and blood.

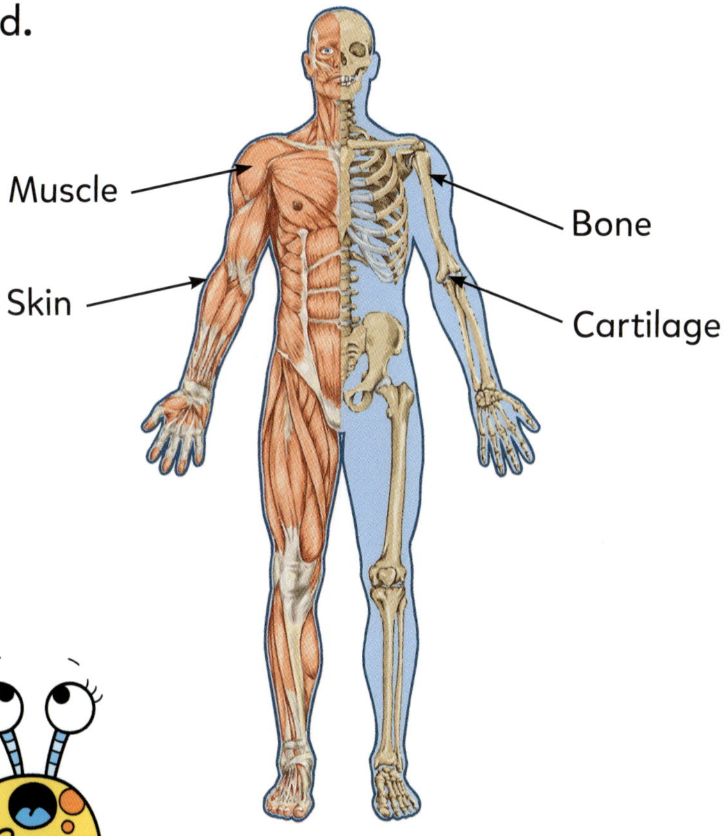

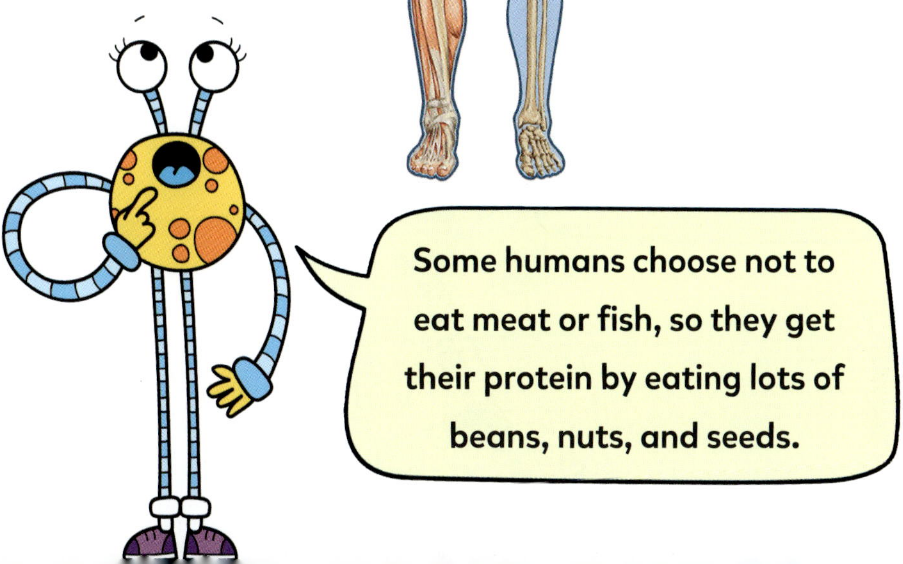

Dairy

Dairy products are good for you because they contain **nutrients** like **calcium.** Calcium makes your bones strong. However, dairy products usually have a lot of fat, so you should watch how much dairy, including milk, butter, and cheese, you eat and drink.

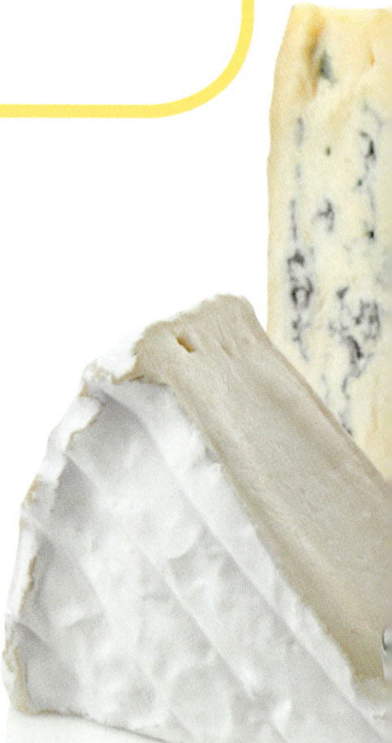

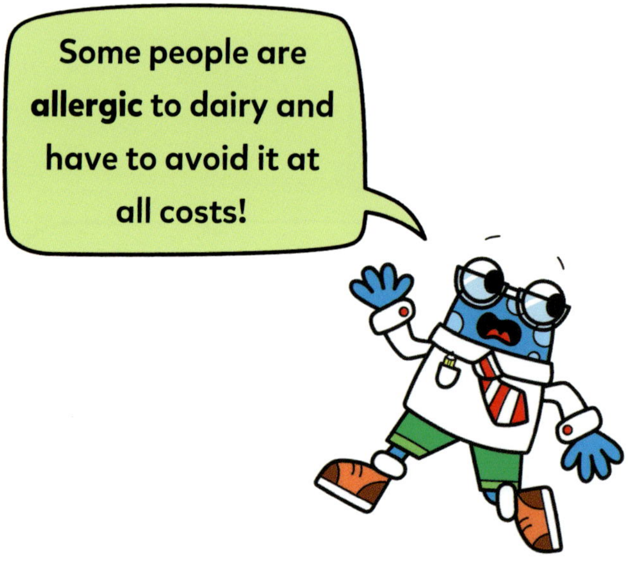
Some people are **allergic** to dairy and have to avoid it at all costs!

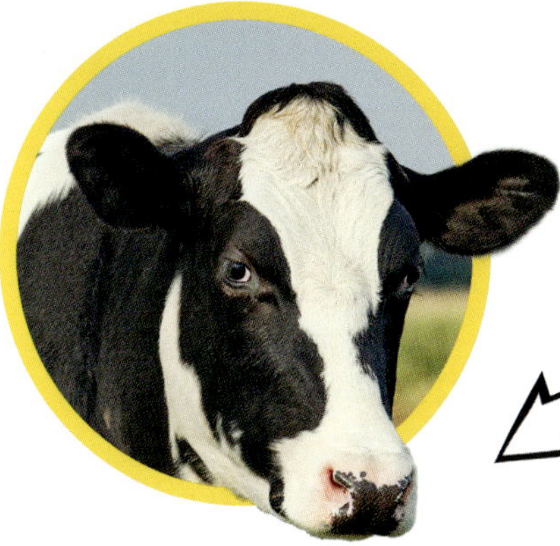

Dairy products are foods made from animal milk, like cows' milk!

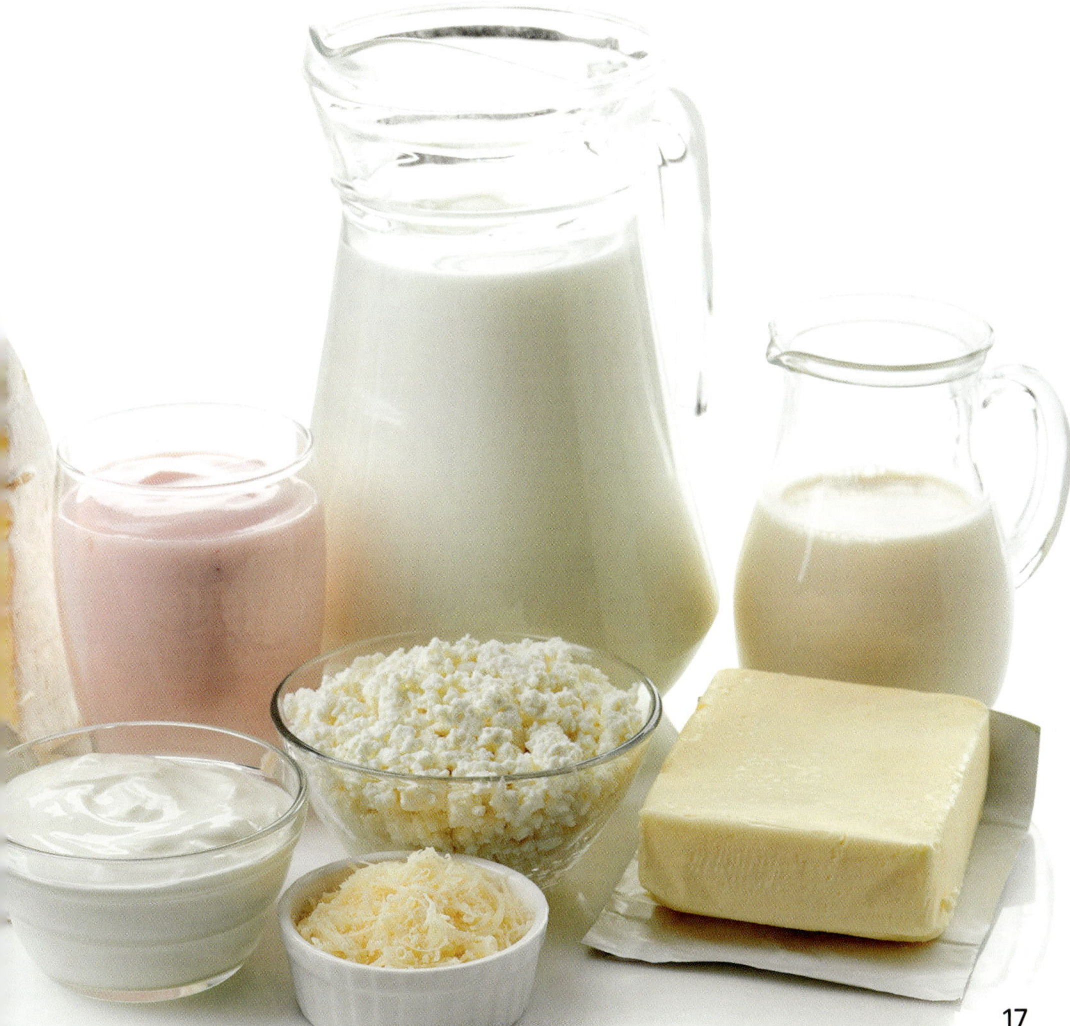

Carbohydrates

Carbohydrates are found in foods such as potatoes, pasta, rice, whole grains, vegetables, fruit, and beans. They are a good source of energy.

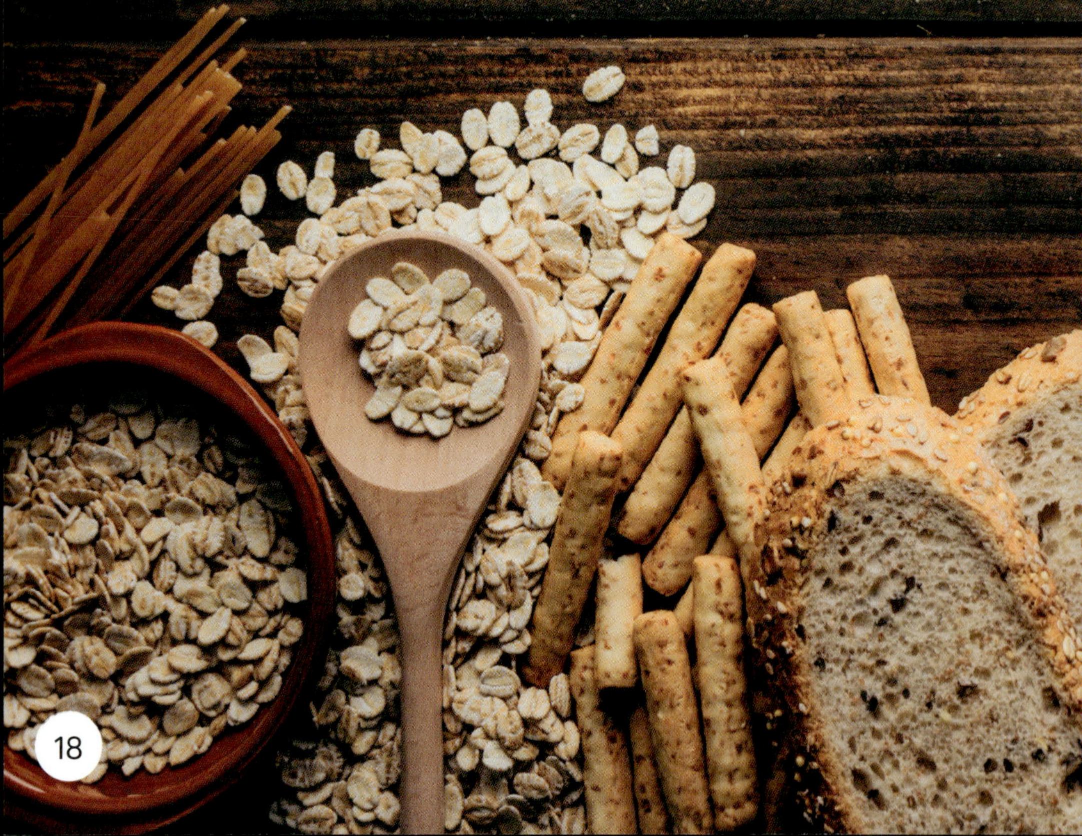

Carbohydrates are good for you, but, like everything else, you have to be careful not to eat too much! Some foods that contain carbohydrates, such as oats and quinoa, are very good for you because they also contain lots of **fiber.**

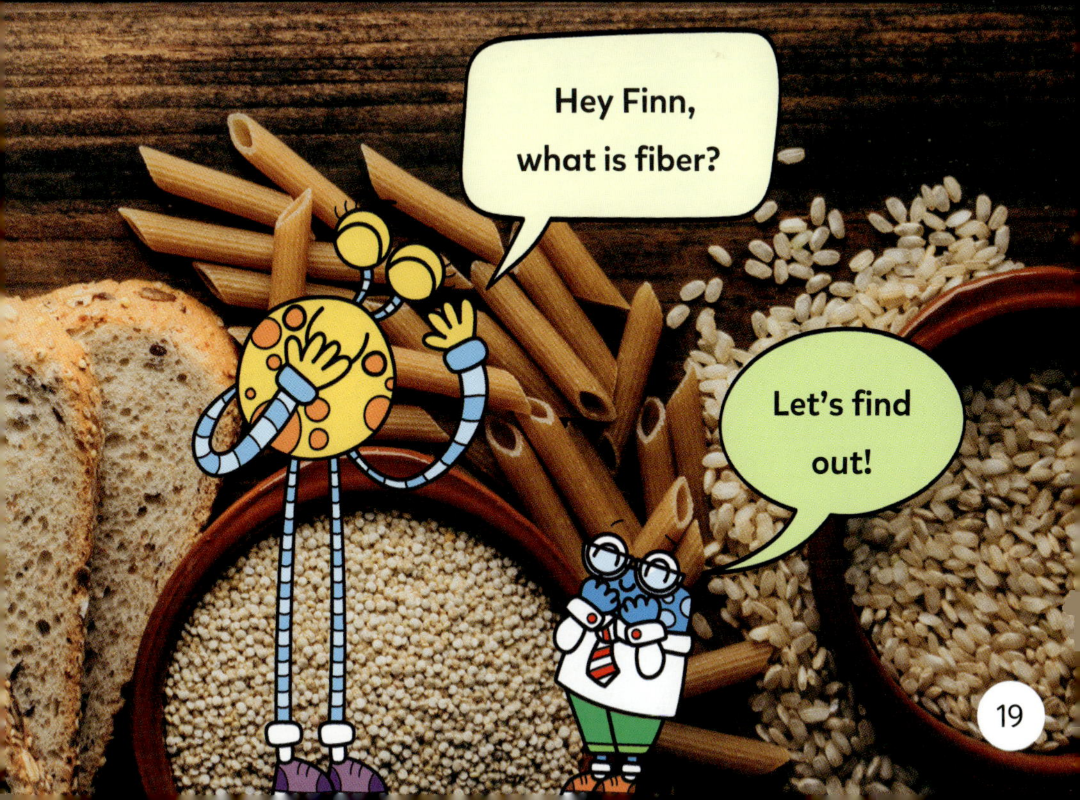

Fiber

Foods that contain lots of fiber help you to feel full. Fiber is good for your **digestion.** Foods with lots of fiber take longer to digest, so you feel full for longer too!

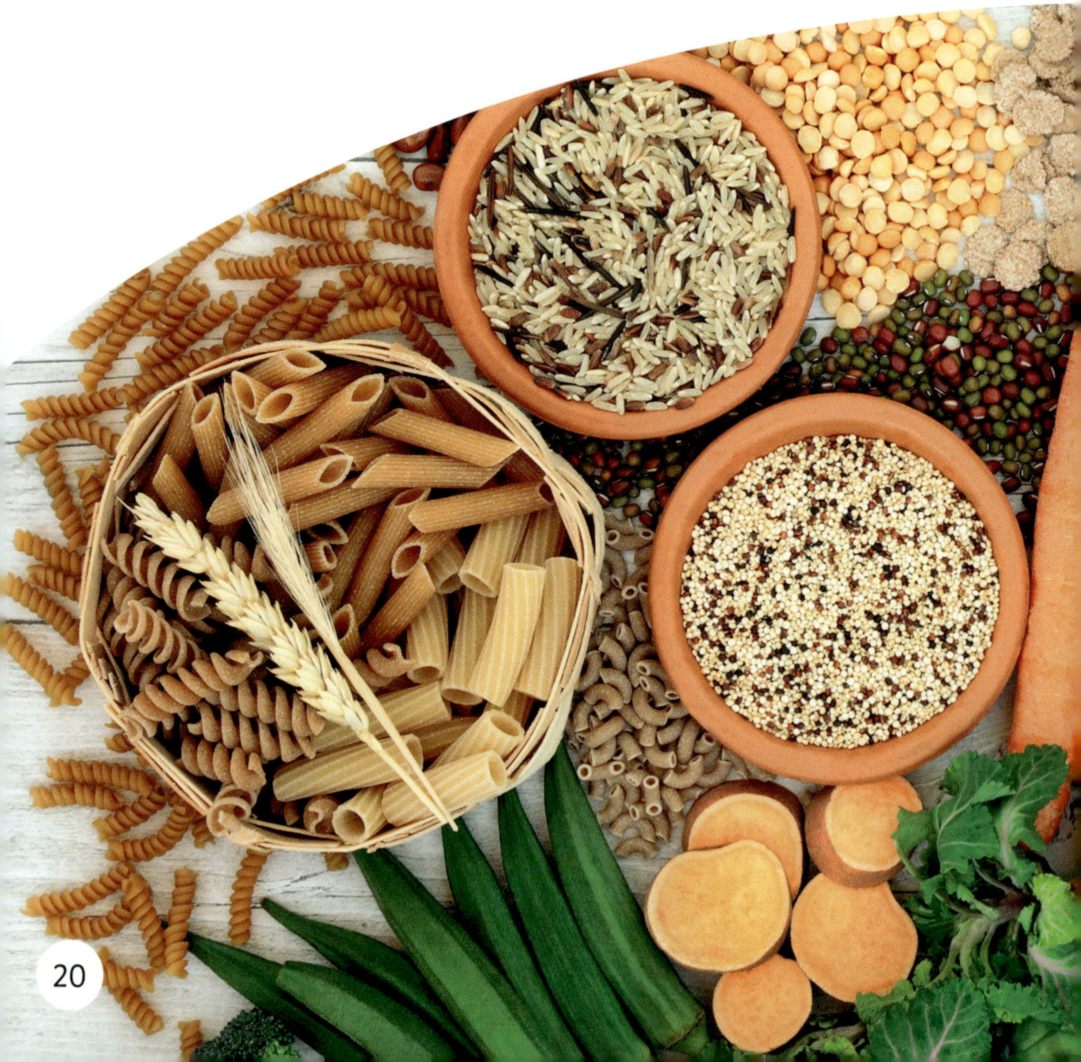

Fiber feeds the good **bacteria** in your **gut.** However, if you eat too much, it can sometimes make you a little gassy!

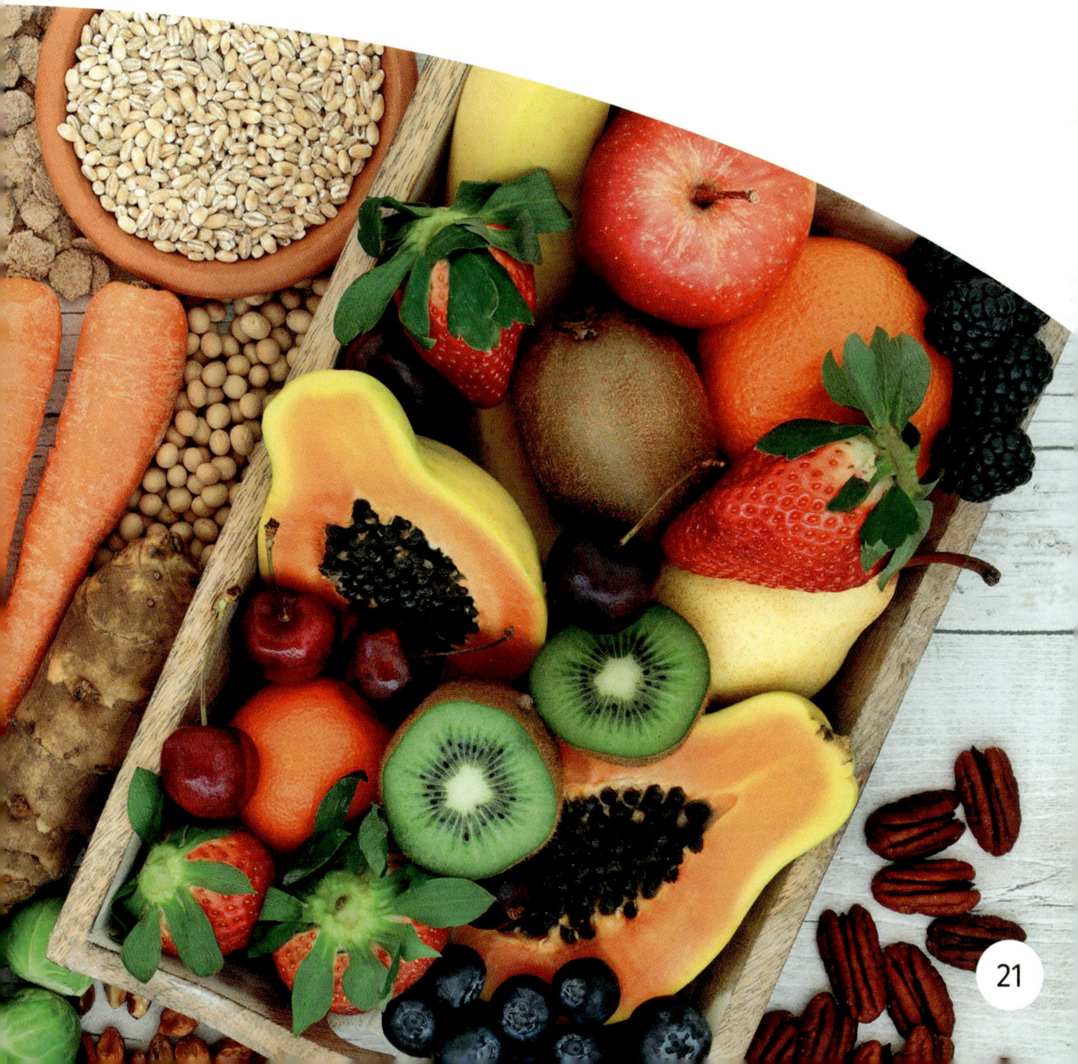

Salt

Salty foods include snacks like fries, chips, pickles, soy sauce, and more!

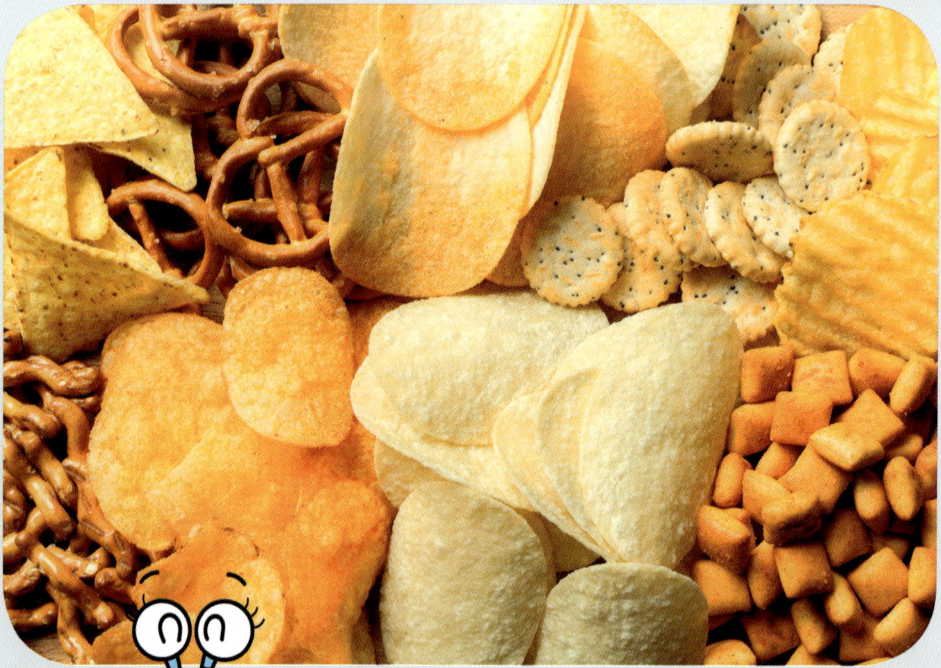

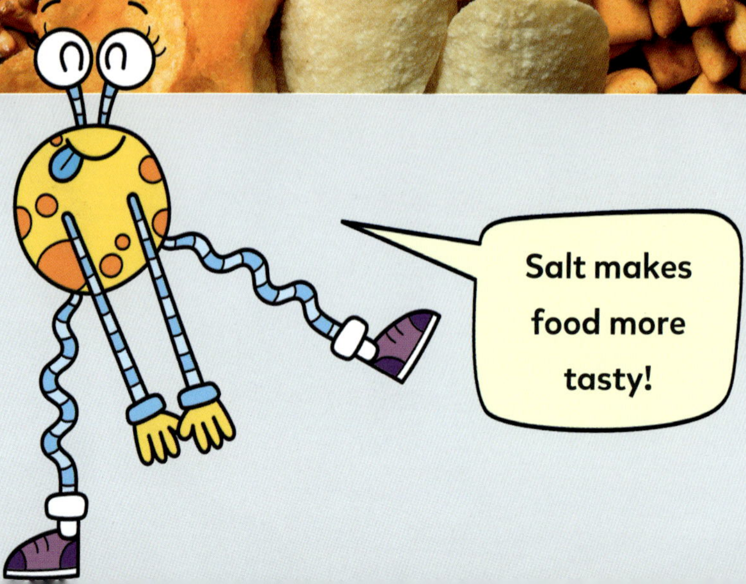

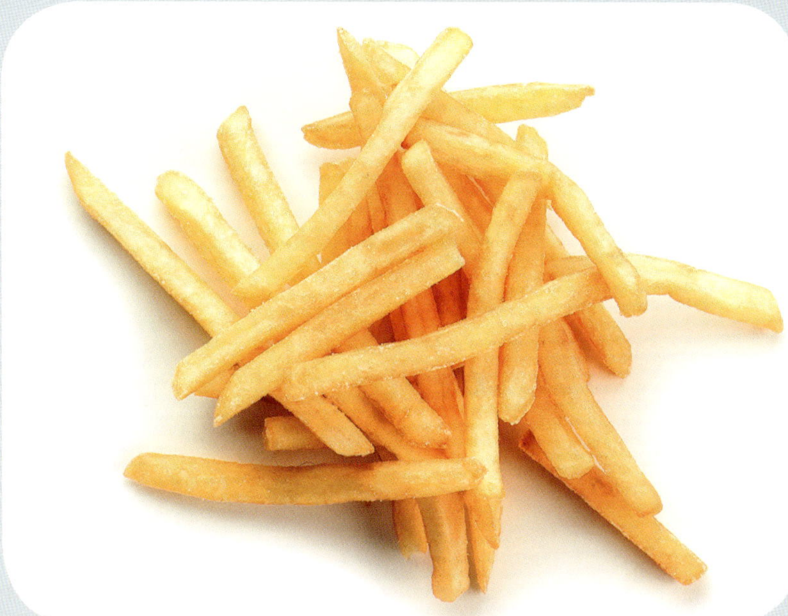

Salt makes your body hold on to water. In the right amounts, salt is very good for you because it contains essential **minerals** that you need to be healthy.

Too much salt can put strain on your heart, kidneys, and brain. It also makes you thirsty!

Vitamins and Minerals

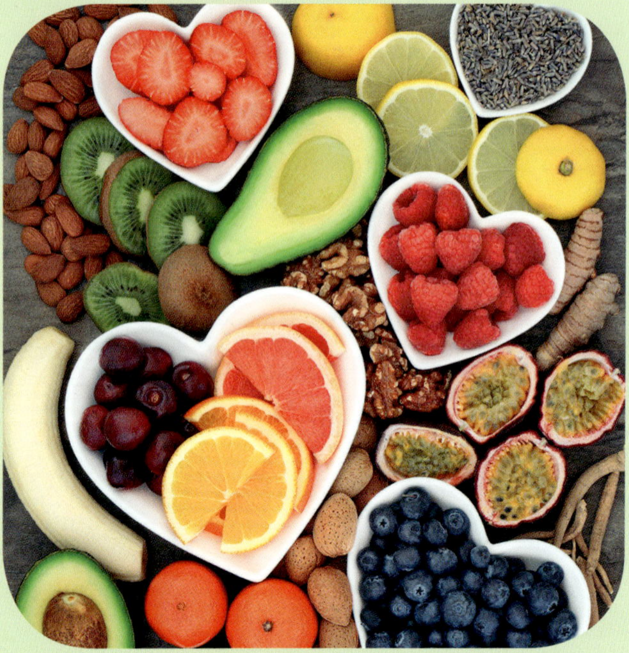

Sailors used to take citrus fruits with them to prevent scurvy, a deadly disease caused by lack of vitamin C!

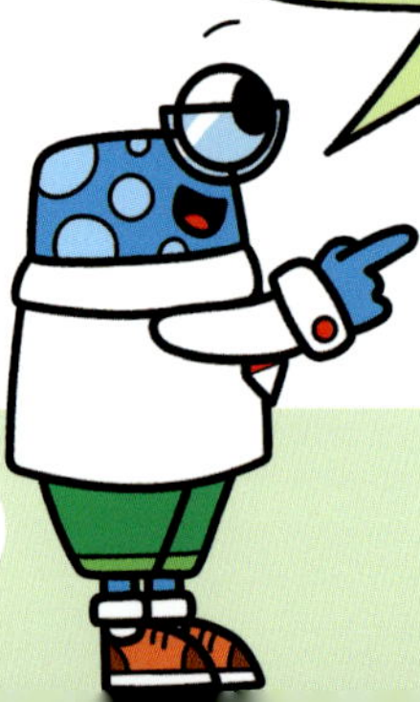

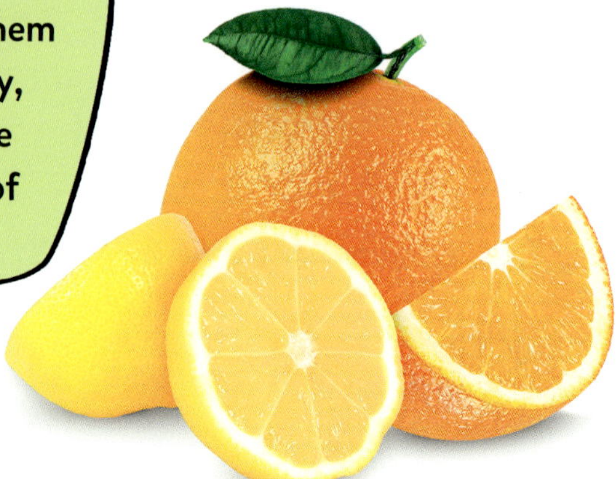

Vitamins and minerals are essential to keep you healthy. Not having enough can be very bad for your body! They can strengthen bones and tissues, help fight colds and flus, keep your skin healthy, and more! Citrus fruits, such as oranges and lemons, are a good source of vitamins and minerals.

Don’t forget to drink plenty of water too!

Water contains minerals and helps the body to work well.

MESSAGE SENT

Dear Om and Nom,

Almost everything humans eat is yummy and good for you, as long as you don't eat too much!

Enjoy tasting lots of different things!

From,
Finn and Zeek

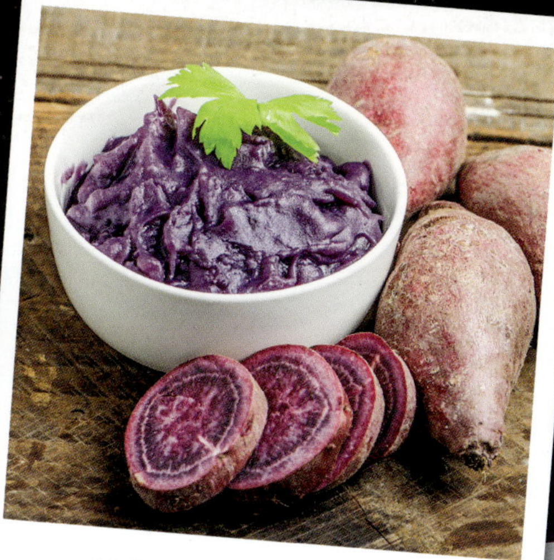

Why not try purple potatoes?

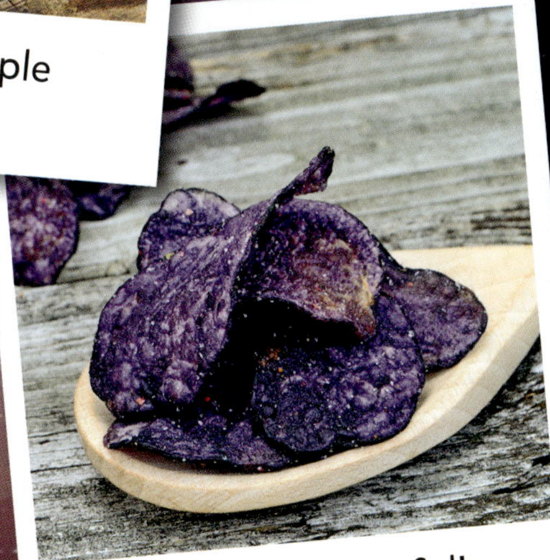

They're so colorful!

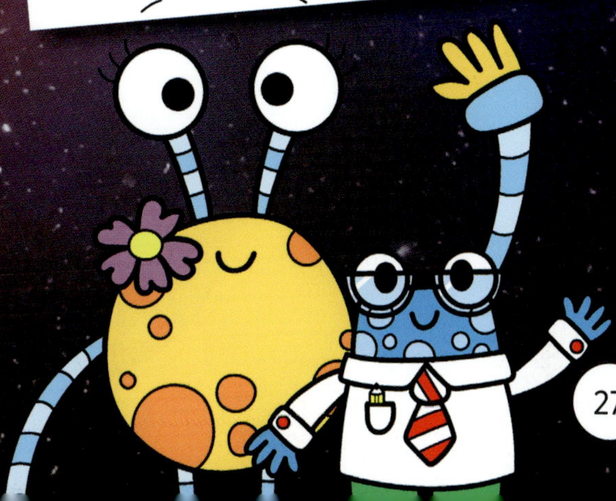

Quiz

1. What kind of diet is best?
   a) One with a lot of fat
   b) One with no sugar
   c) A balanced one

2. What can too much sugar do?
   a) Rot your teeth
   b) Make you healthy
   c) Make you sparkle

3. What food group is animal milk in?
   a) Carbohydrates
   b) Dairy
   c) Fruits

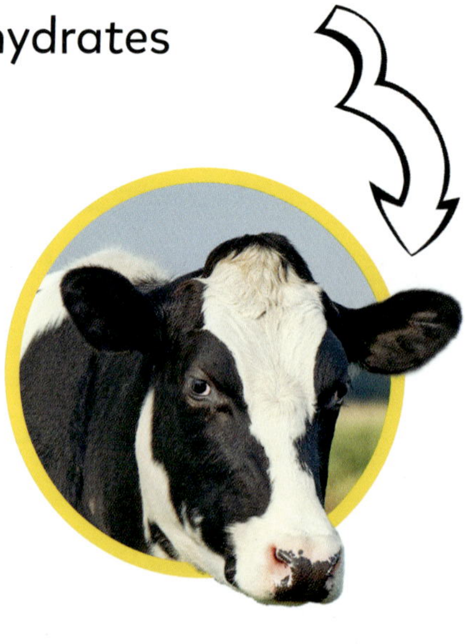

4. Carbohydrates help to . . . ?

   a) Give you energy

   b) Build bones

   c) Store water

5. Which of these foods is salty?

   a) Chocolate

   b) Vegetables

   c) Chips

6. What did sailors take with them to prevent scurvy?

   a) Meat

   b) Citrus fruits

   c) Vegetables

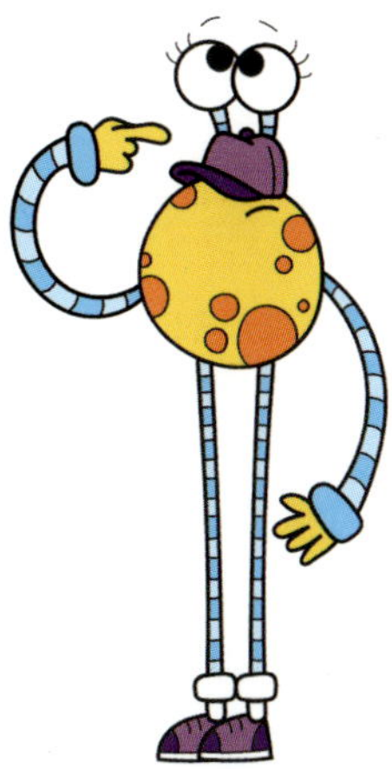

Quiz Answers:
1c, 2a, 3b, 4a, 5c, 6b

Glossary

allergic: having a bad reaction to a particular thing

bacteria: tiny lifeforms made of one cell

calcium: a mineral found in foods and stored in bones and teeth in the body

cartilage: tough, flexible tissue inside the body

digestion: the process that breaks down food, absorbs nutrients, and gets rid of waste

energy: what powers the body and mind

fiber: plant material that can't be digested but that helps you digest other food

gut: stomach

minerals: nutrients that occur naturally in certain foods and that are important for good health

nutrients: substances needed for healthy growth

vitamins: nutrients made by plants and animals

Index

COLOR	GRL
Silver	L-P
Gold	K-L
Purple	J-K
Orange	H-J
Green	G-I
Blue	E-G
Yellow	C-E
Red	C-D
Pink	A-C

Leveled for Guided Reading

Early Bird Stories have been edited and leveled by leading educational consultants to correspond with guided reading levels. The levels are assigned by taking into account the content, language style, layout, and phonics used in each book.

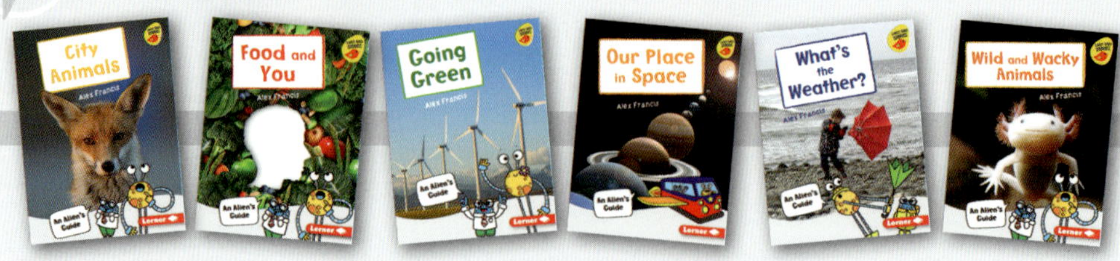